VISION IMPROVEMENT
Secrets

Your Personal Guide To Better Eyes

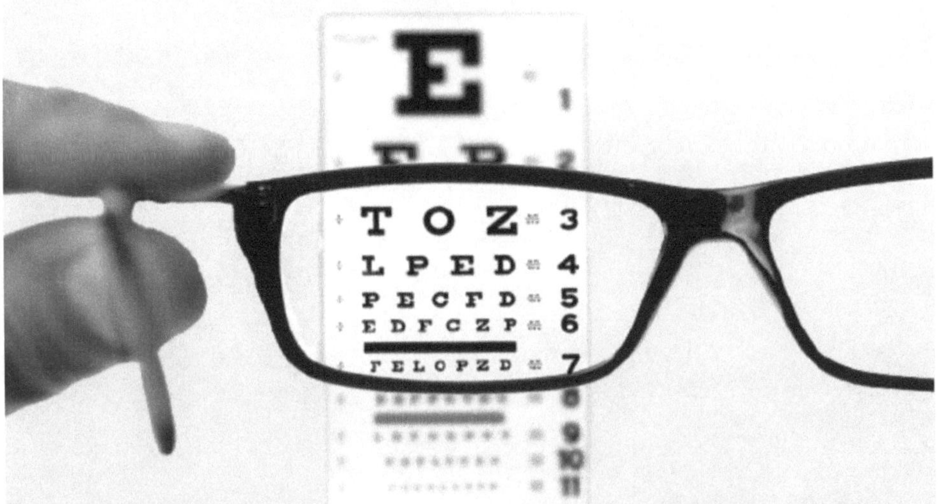

Visible Improvement In 2 Weeks

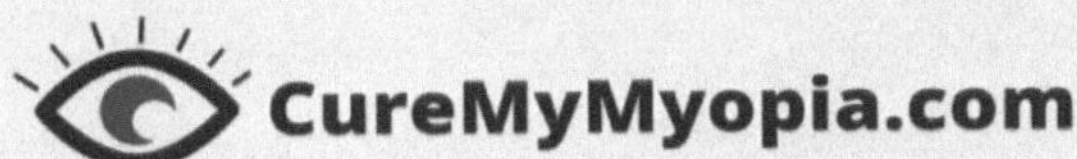

VISION IMPROVEMENT SECRETS

"THE ONLY THING WORSE THAN BEING BLIND IS HAVING SIGHT
BUT POOR VISION."

VISION IMPROVEMENT SECRETS

YOUR PERSONAL GUIDE TO BETTER EYES

© 2021 **CUREMYMYOPIA.COM**

This book is dedicated to all those people
who are suffering from Low vision, Myopia,
Astigmatism, and other eye-related problems.

Contents

WHAT THIS BOOK IS ABOUT?

This book will crush some of the belief systems you will be having about Myopia. This book will show a way to get better eyesight. Not only you will have better eyesight but also will notice a lifestyle change.

You will get to know how myopia is caused and will learn about some terms. You will also get to know how glasses are bad for your eyesight and how bad is Lasik for your eyes.

DISCLAIMER

This information is not intended as a substitute for professional medical advice, emergency treatment, or formal first aid training. Don't use this information to diagnose or develop a treatment plan for a health problem or disease without consulting a qualified health care provider. If you are in a life-threatening or emergency medical situation, seek medical assistance immediately.

Any treatment should be used with utmost precaution and keeping safety in mind. It is very unlikely that the use of any treatment method will cause any harm but if any problem arises then immediately stop the treatment and consult a medical professional. Any advice and treatment should be taken with a grain of salt.

What works for one, may not work for another. The result will vary and will depend on age, health, and other contributory factors. No guarantee could be assured as it is very much subjective and will depend on the efforts and other factors.

The creator/author will not be responsible for any legal action or suit arising out of this guide.

CHAPTER 01

Introduction

What Is Vision Improvement?

For the purposes of this book, vision improvement will be the term used when talking about the process of obtaining clearer vision. There are many different terms used on the Internet and in books, they all mean the same thing, I like vision improvement the best.

Vision improvement is not:

- Squinting to make out the next line on the eye chart
- Wearing pin-hole glasses
- Blinking more/harder/in a funny way to get a different shaped tear film (Contact Effect)
- Doing "eye exercises" or relaxation techniques to get temporary clarity or "clear-flashes"
- This is NOT the Bates Method!

Vision improvement is and can only be:

A long-term, clearer vision that any optometrist can evaluate and verify at any time. It does not require the daily practice of eye exercises. It's permanent. Anything less than this is not worth your time, in the same way, that it wasn't worth mine. Up until very recently, I did not know for sure if this was actually attainable without surgery.

What follows is my own advice, based on my own experience in actually attaining better eyesight.

Before you can go about improving your eyesight, you first have to know how your eyes work. This is the only way to understand how you got duped by all those mainstream optometrists. To do this, we're going to have to dip into clinical science, so just bear with me for a moment.

Pseudomyopia

"You need to wear your glasses at all times in order to keep your vision from getting worse." If this isn't the biggest lie I've ever been told, it's gotta be in the top three at least. The scenario happens every day. A teenager enters an eye doctor's office. An eye exam reveals that their distance vision is fuzzy and they are prescribed glasses. Neither of his or her parents is nearsighted and yet, the eye doctor insists that it's genetics (or a growth spurt) that caused the patient's distance vision to become unsatisfactory. Although it doesn't seem right, the parents accept the verdict, and the teenager gets used to the idea of needing corrective lenses for the rest of their life. The tragedy of the situation is that they didn't need glasses and that glasses will only serve to make their vision worse in the long run. Tragedy, thy name is Pseudomyopia.

Pseudomyopia refers to a passing spasm in the eye's muscles that control focus. There's a circular muscle in your eye that controls the lens and changes shape to give you clear vision at both near and far distances. This is the "ciliary" muscle. When you look at something far away the muscle is relaxed, and when you look at something near the muscle contracts. The closer the point of focus, the greater the contraction in this muscle.

For almost everybody, the first sign of myopia is just a spasm of the ciliary muscle from too much close-up focusing. It's temporary. The muscle locks up and the lens gets **temporarily stuck in the "close-up" mode**. For this reason, you can't see distances clearly. This is pseudomyopia.

First and foremost, pseudomyopia is not my own term, nor is it a term coined by alternative medicine types. Eye doctors of all kinds know this term and understand it completely. It has been scientifically proven. Everyone agrees that it exists and everyone agrees on why it happens.

Pseudomyopia is caused by eyestrain. Not genetics, not

growing eyeballs, none of that.

It's just good ol' too-much-Gameboy or sitting too close to the TV. When an eye doctor finds a patient to be nearsighted, they will prescribe glasses – regardless of the cause. These glasses will have a concave shape (thicker on the outside near the edge, and thinner in the center) and will enable the patient to read the smaller text at a distance while still being able to see up close.

Optically speaking, these glasses work by making distant objects appear closer, and objects close up appear even closer. The problem with prescribing glasses to treat pseudomyopia is that it makes the initial problem worse. Remember that Gameboy screen that was being held too close? Now you're wearing glasses that bring it even closer. By not fixing the initial problem and using a lens that makes the problem even worse, you have accelerated the negative effects. With more eyestrain results, the patient visits the optometrist with worse vision than they had before and leaves with stronger lenses. Within a few years, this vicious cycle will cause the initial pseudomyopia to become real myopia, or what most refer to as axial myopia.

Don't just take my word for it, though. Let's look at a study from the American Academy of Optometry, published back in 1998 and titled, "Vision Therapy to Reduce Abnormal Nearwork-Induced Transient Myopia."

The study followed five subjects with abnormal near-work-induced transient myopia (ANITM) for 7 to 10 weeks as they received vision therapy that utilized tools such as lens flippers and Hart charts. ANITM is a "transient distance blur that is correlated with a transient pseudomyopic shift in…distance refraction" after short periods of near work.

Recordings of subjects' ANITM were taken before and after vision therapy with a Canon R-1 autorefractor, and daily logs were also kept. The study reports that **after therapy, there was marked reduction of symptoms and considerable improvement in clinical accommodative facility measures, as well as** improvement in the objective findings."

Axial Myopia

So you've been going to the eye doctor every 1-2 years just like you were told to. You can no longer function without your glasses or contacts and maybe you're thinking about getting laser corrective surgery. Your driver's license has a letter in the restriction section and when you turn it over it says "corrective lenses." If this is you so far, then I'd like to inform you of your graduation from Pseudomyopia to Axial Myopia.

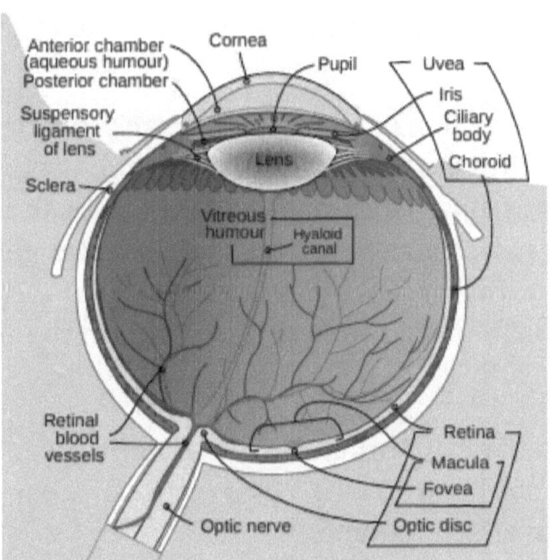

Illustration 1: Cross section view of a human eye.
Source: commons.wikimedia.org

The first thing you should know about normal eyes with 20/20 vision is that they are most comfortable and most relaxed when looking at objects that are 20 feet (or about 6 meters) away or greater. At these distances, light bounces off of the object you're looking at and is scattered in every direction. A small amount of that scattered light gets reflected in your direction, and as science would have it, these rays of light that make it to your eyeballs are traveling parallel to each other. The parallel rays of light pass through the cornea and crystalline lens and are focused on the retina. This creates a clear image that is interpreted by the brain.

So, What Happens When You Look At Something Closer Than 20 Feet?

Light hits the object that you are looking at and is scattered in every direction, just like before. This time, some of the rays of light that make it to your eye are not parallel to each other, they are angled away from each other. The rays of light now pass through the cornea and the lens but do not come to a sharp point of focus on the retina – or at least they wouldn't if the eye's lens couldn't change shape.

The crystalline lens is a flexible sack of clear fluid. It is surrounded by tiny muscle fibers that have the ability to make the front surface of the crystalline lens and the back surface farther apart, thereby making the lens fatter. This changes the angles at which the incoming rays of light are bent and if all goes smoothly, all of the light is focused into a single point on the retina.

To review:

Pseudomyopia: The inability to see distant objects because the ciliary muscle has been strained by overuse of close-up vision. The lens is locked in a fatter shape.

Axial Myopia: A physical response to the conditions of Pseudomyopia. The rear of the eyeball moves back so that light can still be focused on the retina, despite the lens being too fat.

Get it? The eye can see things that are close to it, but it must use small muscle fibers to pull a sack of fluid into a fatter shape. This action, called accommodation, is not easy for the eye to do for long periods of time. If overused, the ciliary muscle will become tired and strained, and will eventually spasm and lock into the flexed position. Distance vision becomes blurry because the lens and ciliary muscle are effectively paralyzed, and the eye is locked in close-up mode. This is the famous "ciliary muscle spasm" which first causes Pseudomyopia, which can become Axial Myopia.

CHAPTER 02

MYTHS

You Have To Always Wear Glasses In Order To Prevent Further Myopia?

How many times you have heard that you have to always wear the glasses or else your vision will decrease. The optometrist also recommends this and this is also a common perception. I want to tell you that this is all B.S, just ask yourself if glasses prevent myopia why you have to change your number frequently. I will tell you how your vision decreases after wearing glasses and lenses.

Your natural eye is the **world's most sophisticated "auto-focus" mechanism**, instantaneously adjusting focus depending on whether you look at something up close, farther away, or very far away. That circular muscle is constantly readjusting to correctly focus light on your retina. It's an amazing system with its constant and instant adjustment of focus.

Glasses, on the other hand, are not so amazing. Your eyes change focal planes dynamically, but glasses do it statically. There is only one adjustment your glasses make, and that goes by whatever diopter number you have. So, glasses do move the light focus (focal plane) inside your eye, just like your natural eye does, but they only do it for one fixed distance.

If you're nearsighted, the lenses are called "minus" lenses. They move the light farther back inside your eye. This compensates for the focusing muscle spasm, but as your eyes adapt to the lenses, **they grow longer**. This is a big topic, the "axial elongation" of your eyeball. Medical science has written hundreds of thousands of pages of studies on this topic.

I'll break it down for you. Your eye isn't this static, dumb thing like the optometrist may make it seem with their static lens corrections. Rather—and hang on to your seat for this—**your eye grows based on what you see around you.**

When you were a baby, you were most likely farsighted (and you probably had astigmatism, too). Then your eye adjusted in length specifically based on its environmental input. It was your vision that determined the axial length of your eyeball (though it's pretty consistent for most people). It's really important to understand that your eye doesn't act independently of the environment.

What you see is truly what you get.

So, if you've ever wondered what causes your prescription to change year after year, this is it. Medical science actually has a word for your ever-increasing myopia: lens-induced myopia (as in, caused by the lenses you wear).

This has been studied over and over, probably in an attempt to find a species for which this doesn't hold true. But any animal's eye that works like ours tends to compensate in the same fashion. Even fish eyes grow longer if minus lenses are put in front of them (don't ask me how they did that). Monkeys (tree shrews?), baby chickens (chicks!), anything and everything gets egg-shaped eyes when minus lenses are used.

If that seems hard to believe, go to Google Scholar (where you can search medical literature) and type in any of the number of terms I've introduced you to pseudomyopia, axial elongation, lens-induced myopia, etc.

But wait a minute. If there are so many studies about this, then why are you still being sold lenses? Well, you're being sold lenses for the same reason I don't want you running off to the optometrist with all this new information to demand answers: There is not some new patented contraption to sell, no branded aspect.

My method isn't going to excite shareholders. It's not going to make profits for some huge corporation, so a lot of the sales-focused outlets aren't exactly going to have a lot of incentive to teach, learn, and practice holistic methods for vision health.

A little side notes: I used to be pretty outspoken against mainstream optometrists, mostly because I looked at them as the enemy. They got me into glasses instead of telling me about prevention. They made a huge profit while my eyes kept getting worse. I was angry about this for many years.

You know what, though? Optometrists are not the enemy at all. They give (most) people what they want: immediate clear vision, regardless of the consequences. You, though, care about those consequences. So, let's get back to your eyes.

You now know the rudiments of how the eye works and how myopia occurs. To break it down in simple terms, though, here are the basic stages of myopia:

1. **Your myopia is a muscle spasm.** Too much close-up work and the muscle gets "locked up" in close-up mode. Distance vision gets slightly blurry.
2. **Minus lenses are offered as therapy.** They move the light farther back in the eye, compensating for the muscle spasm (but not fixing it).
3. **The minus lenses cause the eyes to grow longer.** Now that correction is no longer strong enough (after about a year in the beginning, on average). A higher correction is needed to move the light back farther in the longer eye.

Now, do you see why I developed my method as an alternative to mainstream optometry? Those glasses you're wearing are only contributing to the problem, not solving it.

The single biggest argument made by retail optometry is that the cause of progressive myopia, the axial length of your eyeball, is outside of your control. That's simply not true at all, nothing more than a convenient lie to sell you more glasses.

The same goes for lenses also.

Boggles the mind, doesn't it?

NOW AFTER READING ALL THIS, I DON'T WANT YOU TO THROW YOUR EYEGLASSES.

What I want from you is to reduce your glasses number. You will get to know about differential glasses and Diopter reduction in **Treatment 2**.

Lasik Is An Instant Fix And Safe Also?

You would probably be thinking Lasik is an instant fix and is so cheap now. It's only $300/$200/10- cents per eye and it only takes 15 minutes. Why would I waste my time on this? "

How do you feel about gastric bypass? Even surgeons who perform it know that it's no substitute for a good-old-fashioned diet and exercise. This is what we're talking about here, diet and exercise versus weight loss surgery. If you want a better analogy, this is gastric bypass versus weight loss by buying smaller clothes.

Lasik is not worth any amount of money because it's not a real solution to the problem. Lasik does not decrease the axial length of the eye and thus does not reduce the risk of retinal detachment. Lasik, Lasek, and PRK work by carving the surface of the eye (cornea) into a permanent contact lens.

There is no guarantee that you will walk away with 20/20 vision, or even 20/40. Many people need repeat "touch up" sessions and the FDA has considered outlawing it in the United States. Read the FDA study on Lasik sometime, it's a real hoot.

CHAPTER 03

TREATMENTS

Pseudomyopia Treatment

Let's say you or your child are experiencing blurry distance vision. Maybe they only notice after playing Gameboy for 2 hours straight or yourself after working on those TPS reports all night long. You just received the note from the school nurse, glasses have not been prescribed yet, you're thinking about going to the optometrist soon. Don't bother.

All you have to do is use your distance vision. Go outside for a walk and look at those fuzzy letters on license plates and street signs. Stay in and watch a movie with the subtitles on. Make it a foreign film.

Just do something that requires you to look at something 15-20 feet away for a while. Do this every day and you'll be back to 20/20 in a few weeks.

Practice the 20/20/20 rule. You have proven to yourself that you are prone to giving yourself Pseudomyopia through bad habits, so the obvious solution is to get a good habit. When looking at things close up for extended periods of time, take a break every 20 minutes, focus on something at least 20 feet away for at least 20 seconds. That's it. No eye yoga, no supplements, no surgery, and no glasses.

You can stop reading here.

Axial Myopia Treatment

You went to the eye doctor and started wearing glasses sometime between last year and thirty-five years ago. Don't worry, so did I. The solution isn't as easy to explain or as fast-acting as the one for Pseudomyopia, but it does work for everyone and in my opinion, it's the only real solution.

You can wear glasses or contacts, or go get laser surgery but none of that will reduce the axial length of the eye and decrease your risk of a detached retina. First and foremost, anybody out there who says "you can restore your natural vision naturally as nature natured it in 10 natural minutes/days/seconds" is a big fat liar. Ever see an infomercial for exercise equipment? They spend just as much time talking about how easy it's going to be to get sixpack-abs as they talk about the actual product that they're selling. This is going to take months, or years. Progress will be slow, but measurable. In order to be successful, you will need to make this a (small) part of your daily life.

Let me put it to you like this: you've been wearing glasses for X amount of years, your prescription has gotten worse and worse. If you could reverse that process of worsening vision by putting a small amount of effort every day and it would take less than X number of years, would you do it?

That's all I promise and nothing more. I wore glasses for 12 years, my vision became progressively worse as the prescriptions became stronger. I reversed the process and my vision became better and better. I undid the damage caused by 12 years of bad habits and bad glasses in less than one year. Imagine being able to look at your own clear reflection in the mirror and know that you fixed the problem yourself. It's so worth it.

So, let's get started...

TREATMENT 1

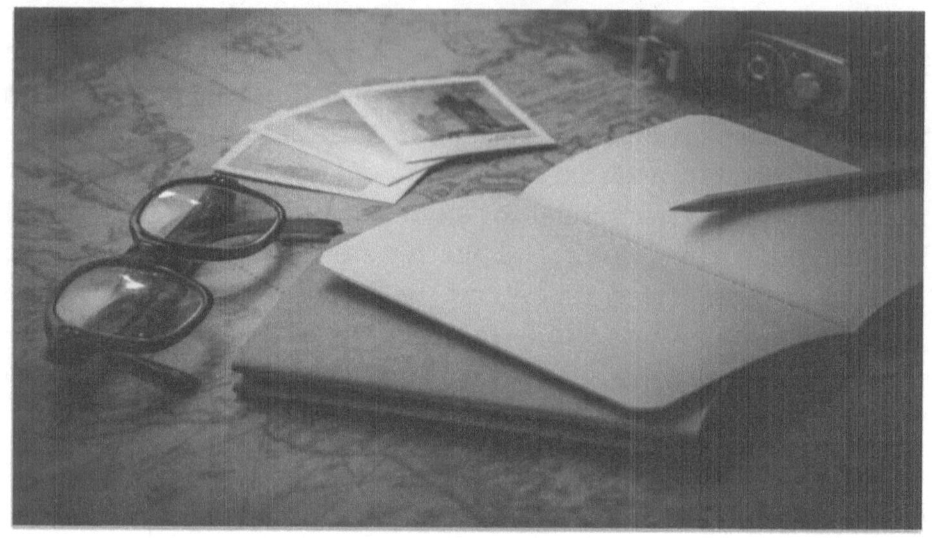

THE ANCIENT METHOD

Introduction

The human system is designed to treat itself. Our wounds start automatically healing after some time. So does our eyesight. If we stop doing close-up work, our eyesight will start going back to normal.

In earlier times there were no eyesight problems because there were no smartphones, TV, laptops. But in today's times, most of our work involves close-up screen work. Staying away from the screen is very difficult. The only way we can improve our eyesight is by introducing some lifestyle changes.

Follow this guide thoroughly and apply all the information that is given.

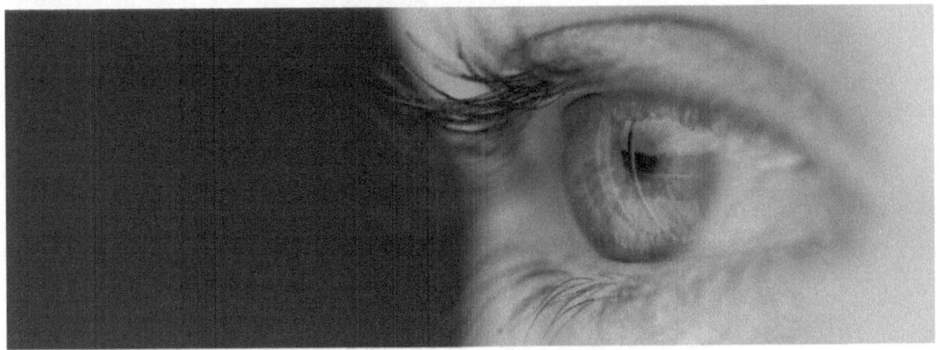

Ever thought about how animals treat their wounds? They don't have access to medicines or any lab-developed ointments. They use their saliva to treat the wounds, cuts.

Cuts and wounds in our mouth heal faster than similar cuts and wounds anywhere else on our body. Scientists were astonished by this information and they started conducting different experiments. They wanted to test the healing property of saliva.

They scraped the epithelial cells layers and placed them in Petri dishes. The cells were then wounded by scrapping a small piece of the cell layer away. Some of the cells were treated with saliva and the other with an isotonic solution. The discovery surprised the scientist as the cells that were treated with saliva closed after 16 hours while the other cells that were treated with isotonic solutions were still open. It was strong evidence that saliva accelerated the healing process.

The component that was responsible for this accelerated healing was identified as **Histatin.**

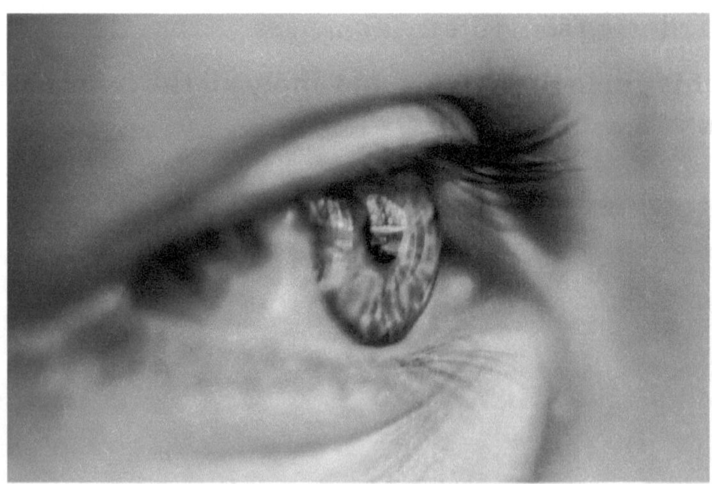

Now the question arises how we can use our saliva to cure our eyesight? As gross as it may sound but this is how people use to treat their eyesight earlier. This knowledge was long lost.

Hundreds of people benefited from using this method. Don't believe me, just use this method for 2 months and find out yourself. This is one of the fastest and low-maintenance methods.

You don't have to buy anything. It may look gross but if it can help you get clear eyesight then you should give it a try.

You can try other methods that I have provided but believe me this is the best method. When I started using this method I was able to see visible changes in 1 week. It may vary from person to person. One of my clients was able to cure his myopia of -1.75 using this method in only 55 days.

Points To Remember Before Starting This Method

- Only Morning saliva is to be used.
- You should not drink water and not even brush your teeth before trying this method.
- This should be the first thing you should do after waking up.
- You Should have good oral health.
- You have to brush 2 times a day using chemical-free toothpaste.
- Brushing at night time is mandatory.
- Don't forget to clean your tongue.
- You have to keep your body hydrated.

Method

- Firstly, maintain good oral health. If your oral health is not good don't proceed with this method, try another method. If you have any mouth infection or other oral problems don't proceed. You have to keep your body well hydrated so that it can produce good saliva.
- Start by brushing at night and waking up in the morning. Don't drink water or anything and don't even brush. Now take your saliva in your hand and apply it to your eyes like a kajal (apply on your lower eyelid). You can search on Google "How to apply Kajal".
- After applying the saliva just close your eyes for 10-15

min. After that open your eyes and now you can proceed with your daily routine. Try to wash your eyes after 1 hour only to have the maximum result.

- Only do this method one time in the morning. Don't repeat it because saliva is not very effective afterward as after eating food, saliva is contaminated and can cause problems or infection in the eye.

Things To Do While Following The Method

- Try To have good oral health. Clean your tongue and teeth properly. If you have any oral problems then visit a dentist and after that only follow this method.
- Have a good sleeping schedule and a good and timely diet.
- Try this method at least for a minimum of 2 months and then only have an eye test.
- Try to use your eyeglasses as little as possible. If you have myopia don't use your eyeglasses for close work. Only use it when you really need it like for driving.
- Limit your screen time. Don't use mobile for long and also limit your laptop usages.
- Play outdoor games and go walking.
- Instead of using mobile, go for a long walk and look at greenery, signboards, etc.
- Challenge your eyesight by looking at distant objects.

TREATMENT 2

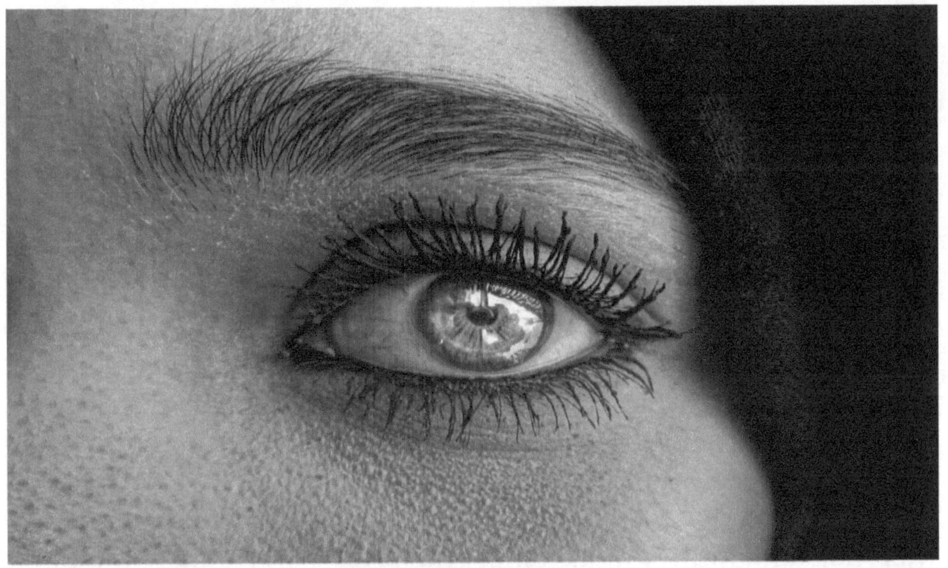

ACTIVE FOCUS

Lesson One: Ever-Changing Optics And The Theory Of Vision Improvement.

Get some reading material and remove your glasses. Get close enough to see the text crystal clear. Move the text away until the letters just start to become fuzzy and hold it there. Really look at each individual letter, notice the nuances of the font and the spacing between each character. After a time (usually less than a minute) you'll notice that the fuzzy text became clearer without moving closer.

Here's what's happening: Your eyes and your brain work together. The brain knows what the letter T looks like and when the eye sends a signal to the brain that says "fuzzy T," the brain knows that something is wrong. Ultimately it is the brain that controls all aspects of the eye, including those tiny muscles that pull on the lens. If you couldn't get the text to become clear or cannot repeat it, don't worry.

What we're trying to do here is get the brain (specifically, the visual cortex) to understand that the image is wrong. I'm familiar with one scientific study which showed that this eyeball-brain combination can figure out not only that the image is blurry but also, how and why the image is blurry. It is the exact same mechanism that made your eyesight become worse in the first place.

What Glasses Do To The Eyes And Visual Cortex

It confuses them. Wearing glasses that improve distance vision, to look at things up close confuses the eyes and visual cortex (brain) into adjusting for Hyperopia (farsightedness).

Picture this: you're 12 years old in school and you're furiously writing that essay portion of your mid-term exam. Under the stress, you keep moving your face closer and closer to the piece of paper that you're writing on. Each time you move closer to the paper, the lines and writing become just a little bit blurry. This is a hyperopic blur. Then the blurriness resolves into clarity. This is caused by the brain and eyes engaging in a kind of troubleshooting game. The brain sees the signs of farsightedness and says to the eyes,

"More accommodation! Fatter lens!"

The eyes reply, "Accommodation is at 70 percent, increasing to 80 percent."

"That's good. Clear image sighted. Hold it there."

You move closer to the paper, the brain sees the text go out of focus again in the hyperopia direction.

"Fatter lens!" The brain demands.

This process repeats until the eyes finally answer, "We've given it all we've got!

Accommodation levels are critical! 101 percent!"

At this, the brain barks, "Emergency maneuvers! Increase axial length!" and the whole eye becomes longer.

Thus, the entire theory behind vision improvement is to stimulate the eyes with opposite conditions from the ones detailed above, in order to achieve the opposite and desirable effect.

Lesson Two: How To Stimulate The Eyes Into Improving

Consider what we've learned so far:

- A normal eye is most relaxed while focusing on

something 20 feet away or greater.
- The eye has a flexible lens that enables it to focus on things closer than 20 feet.
- When the ciliary muscle is relaxed, the (crystalline) lens is flat and the eye is brought to (normally infinite) distance focus.
- Minus lenses prescribed to correct nearsightedness work by making things closer and smaller, as viewed through the lenses.
- Viewing objects close up requires the eyes to focus on a blurry image. The eyes and brain can figure out WHY the image is blurry (it's too close) and HOW to bring it into focus (accommodation and then increase the axial length).

We have established that the eyes and brain recognize two different types of blur. Borrowing the terms used in the cited study, we will call them,

Myopic Defocus: caused by objects being too far away. Think, blurry chalkboard.

Hyperopic Defocus: caused by objects being too close. Think, a toddler showing you something by holding it 2 inches in front of your eyes.

Hyperopic defocus occurs just before accommodation, so as long as that works properly, we never even see it. The eyes refocus too fast to see the blurry image. However, we do feel the aftereffect in the form of eyestrain, which is the strain of actual muscle doing actual work. Hyperopic defocus is balanced by myopic defocus, which is the signal for the ciliary muscle to relax and for axial length to decrease.

In short, the very symptom that brought you to the eye doctor in the first place, when you couldn't read the chalkboard, is what is necessary to stimulate the eyes into decreasing axial length.

You need to subject your eyes to myopic defocus while

reducing, but not eliminating their exposure to hyperopic defocus. Simply put, you need to do 2 things:

1. See a small amount of blurriness in the distance by reducing your distance prescription.
2. Be mindful of how much time you spend looking at things that are close up.

A Word On Astigmatism

Before We get to talking about specific vision improvement plans, I need to explain how astigmatism is notated on your prescription and how it relates to reduced lens therapy.

	Sphere	Cylinder	Axis
O.D.	-1.75	-0.25	100
O.S.	-1.50		

On your eyeglasses prescription, there should be two main rows, OD and OS, these stand for your right and left eyes, respectively. These two rows are then divided into 3 columns, Sphere (Sph), Cylinder (cyl), and Axis. The last two are for astigmatism (cylinder and axis). Simplifying here, Astigmatism is when the surface of the eye or cornea, is not a perfect, regular-shaped sphere, it curves more on one axis (say, north-south) than the other axis (east-west).

I hate this analogy but I have no choice but to use it: picture an (American) football. The cylinder number is how inflated the football is and the axis number is its orientation.

When Ordering A Pair Of Glasses, Follow These Rules For Astigmatism:

- If you've only got a -0.75, -0.50 or -0.25 in the cylinder column, don't bother with the next steps. Order your

> glasses with the cylinder and axis boxes blank.

- Astigmatism can be corrected by increasing the sphere value by 50% of the cylinder value. For example, you've got a -3.00 sphere, -1.00 cylinder, axis 100, change it to -3.50 sphere, BLANK cylinder, axis BLANK. This is called a spherical equivalent.
- You do not have to use a spherical equivalent, you can reduce the cylinder value incrementally if you wish. If you go that route, keep the axis value the same.
- Remember, this is not rocket science. So long as you don't change the numbers too much, you can't go wrong. Worst case scenario, you wind up ordering a pair of glasses that make you feel uncomfortable – which isn't a big deal since most sites have a no-questions-asked replacement policy.

Once again. Reduced lens therapy is not rocket science. Do not get scared away by this stuff. Reduce the sphere and cylinder values on your prescription in small steps, and your eyes will improve. It's really that simple. Seriously, you could stop reading here if you wanted.

Obtaining Weaker Glasses

Guess what? You're now your own optometrist. That guy or gal in the white coat probably isn't going to cooperate with this stuff. The good news is, you can order your own glasses online without a prescription (they're not even real prescriptions in the first place), and it's a piece of cake. My favorite site for this is eyebuydirect but zennioptical is also good. I've used both and had a great experience every time.

Basically, you go on the site, pick out frames (you can upload a photo of your face to try them on and approximate the size), enter the prescription and options for coatings (get the anti-glare/antireflective, trust me, you'll want it) and then it's just like buying anything else on the Internet. Shipping address, payment, and done.

When you get this first pair of glasses, take note of sizing information on the product page for that specific frame. Write it down and keep your own record of it. You may find that you hit the nail on the head with the first pair and you'll want the sizing info for the next pair. These sites often have useful measurements that aren't in the standard sizing info on the frame itself, and they change out inventory periodically. You may try to look up your frame to see how the hinge to hinge measurement compares to a prospective new frame only to find that they discontinued the frame and that precious data is gone. Ask me how I know this.

How frame sizing works: it's 3 numbers, such as 53-19-141 (my size) which correspond to the width of one of the lenses (53mm on mine), the width of the nose piece (19mm), and the overall length of one of the frame's arms (141mm).

If you're at all scared by the prospect of figuring out your own prescription and ordering your own glasses, ask yourself, what's the worst that can happen? You're eyes get screwed up and your vision gets worse? Newsflash, that's already happening under the supervision of an optometrist. They have failed to help you. If you want something done right, you do it yourself.

Now, let's get started with the treatment.

Prerequisites

You will need:

1. A Snellen eye chart. Buy one online (eBay, Amazon, etc...) or print one out from http://www.i-see.org/ eyecharts
2. A copy of your eyeglass prescription
3. A do it yourself attitude and persistence

Action Plan 1: Starting From High Myopia

Your prescription has numbers greater than 6 (-6.00, -7.00, etc...) in the Sph (sphere) column. Your eye doctor talks to you in somber tones about the risk of retinal detachment but hasn't told you what to do about it.

Here's what you do about it:

- Set up an eye chart either in good lighting indoors or in the shade outdoors. Look at it from 20 feet away with your glasses on.
- If you can see better than the 40-foot line (20/40), obtain weaker glasses (see the relevant section). You're going to want to lower the values in the sphere column on your current prescription by 1 whole diopter. For example, if you're at a -7.00 in one eye and a -7.75 in the other, lower it to -6.00 and -6.75, respectively.
- If you can only just barely make out the letters on the 40-foot line, keep your current glasses until you can see the 32ft line (one below).
- Wear these less-than-20/40 glasses whenever it is not critical that you have perfect distance vision, such as doing laundry, watching TV, work, etc... Do not wear them while say, driving at night or vampire hunting.
- Test your vision in these new glasses periodically using the eye chart. When you can see better than 20/40, repeat the process from step 2. When your prescription is reduced to fewer than 6 diopters, move on to the next section.

Action Plan 2: Moderate Myopia

The sphere column has numbers that are less than 6 but greater than 2.

- Perform the same process as Action Plan 1: eye chart, test vision...
- This time, when it's time to lower your prescription it's

going to be in smaller steps. Here's the sequence: -6.00 →
-5.00 → -4.50 → - 4.00 → -3.50 → -3.00 → -2.75 → -2.50 →
-2.25 → -2.00

- Notice that these are +1.00 steps, to begin with, then +0.50, and finally +0.25, which is the smallest increment that you can change the lens power by. If you'd like to know why to look at the handy table in the appendix at the end of the book.
- Same as before, lower the prescription when you can see better than 20/40.

Action Plan 3: Mild Myopia, The Final Stretch

Your prescription is less than 2.00 Diopters.

- Perform the same process as Action Plan 1: eye chart, test vision...
- When it's time to reduce the prescription, reduce it in steps of 0.25 (unfortunately, this is the smallest increment, see appendix).
- If you've gotten to this stage from moderate or high myopia, be prepared for this part to take a very long time.

Optional For All 3 Plans And A Word On Positive Lens Usage.

- For best results, order another pair of glasses for close-up stuff, such as reading or working on a computer. Do this by adding +1.25 to your distance prescription for computer work and +2.50 for reading. For example, if you've got a -6.00 then, -6.00 + 1.25 = -4.75
- If you follow this process and reduce your prescription down to -2.00, or if you start at -2.00 (or less) you have a decision to make. Watch this: -2.00 + 2.50 (for reading) = +0.50

Do You Want To Use A Positive Lens For Close-Up Stuff?

This is usually referred to as positive lens therapy. I heard a story somewhere that during World War II there were recruits who wanted to be pilots but couldn't pass the vision test. These enterprising recruits somehow figured out that if they wore weak reading glasses (positive lenses, such as +1.00) for a small amount of time, their uncorrected distance vision would permanently improve. I have been unable to fact-check this story but it would make sense and it would actually work. However, though I did find that my own distance vision improved when I used positive lenses in the form of reading glasses, there are two considerations that caused me, to discontinue their use.

1. **Presbyopia:** we lose our ability to accommodate as we age. Every second that you use a positive lens to see up close, your lens is flat and not flexing. It may be the case that you use it or lose it.

2. **Accommodation and Convergence:** In their natural state, the eyes have a shortcut for focusing on close-up objects. As an object gets closer, the eyes have to converge or turn toward one another. The eyes and brain learn that there is an amount of accommodation that matches this convergence. Unfortunately, looking through corrective lenses will disrupt this process and alter the amount of accommodation needed. It has already been screwed up by wearing distance glasses, do you really want to screw it up more with reading glasses?

Bottom line: I continued to improve despite my decision to avoid positive lenses and really, I wanted to improve my vision so that I could be free of glasses. Why introduce more glasses into my life?

That's it

That's everything you need to know in order to reverse your progressing myopia through reduced lens therapy, and I even explained positive lens therapy, despite not recommending it. You can go out on the Internet and pay for all sorts of books and memberships to forums, but you're not going to find anything beyond what I've written here that will actually help you to improve your vision. Trust me, I've looked and I've tried everything.

The B Word

"But..."

"...I heard that all you have to do is perform these simple exercises every day and get better vision."

So these eye exercises, do you do them with glasses on or off? How do you know if you're doing them correctly? Why isn't necessary for people with normal vision to do these exercises? Why isn't there anyone out there with cold, hard, objective proof of vision improvement through eye exercises? They may work for some people, but it's my opinion that they are unnecessary. Animal studies showed that vision worsened and then improved in response to lens usage and reduction. I'm pretty sure they didn't make the chickens and marmosets do eye exercises. Same with the human study

"...I like wearing my glasses. They're fashionable/make me look cute/distract from my humpback/etc..."

You can use these techniques to reduce your dependence on glasses by reducing your prescription or just to stop your vision from getting worse. You don't have to rid yourself of glasses completely, just get out of harm's way (retinal detachment) or get rid of your coke-bottle lenses.

"...going to the optometrist and getting new glasses is too expensive. What am I supposed to do, go there every month when my vision improves?"

Nope. Do it yourself. You're fully capable of looking at an eye chart from 20 feet away and typing a few numbers into an order form. You can get a complete pair of glasses online for $20 including shipping and everything, or a really nice pair of glasses for $40.

"...ordering my own glasses is way too hard and I can't figure out the prescription."

Really it's not. Just try it. You'll figure it out. If you really can't do it and you're stumped, contact me. Seriously, I don't bite and I'll take the 30 seconds to write back. You're really not putting me out by asking.

Questions And Answers

Q: Let's say a person has mild myopia and they've never worn glasses. Why do they have bad vision and why doesn't their vision improve?

A: Their vision is bad because they have bad habits, such as looking at a smartphone 6 inches from their face for hours at a. If you don't change the habit, vision doesn't improve.

Q: Why can't I just take off my glasses and have a better vision? stretch

A: You can, but most people don't like to be blind. If you have just a little bit of blur, you'll have a totally functional vision and still improve. It's the best of both worlds.

Q: Is there a way to improve my vision while wearing contacts?

A: Possibly. I've never worn contacts for that much time, so I don't feel qualified to recommend a plan of improvement that uses contacts instead of glasses.

Q: I only have astigmatism, will this stuff work for me?

A: Yes, make the numbers on your prescription smaller (don't change the axis value) and order the glasses. I dare to say that astigmatism is more lens-induced than myopia.

Q: What about print pushing?

A: Print pushing is the most common name for the practice of placing text at a distance where it just starts to become blurry and then adjusting the distance so that the text goes from blurry to clear. After practicing this, you will notice that the point at which the text becomes blurry is further than it used to be. This is good.

Practice print pushing in 15-minute sessions, twice per day but don't try too hard to make the blurry text clearer. This will strain your eyes and make your vision worse.

Q: I have two different eyes (Anisometropia), one's worse than the other. Will this work for me?

A: Yes. I have 2 different refractive errors. What you want to do is get the prescriptions to be equal but don't make drastic changes. IE. Go for -2.00,-2.00 instead of -2.50,-2.00 Do not go from -3.00,-2.00 to -2.00, -2.00

Q: I (or someone I know) have worn glasses my whole life but recently my prescription decreased instead of increase like normal. Why is that?

A: When I hear this question it's usually from people who are about 30-40 years of age. My theory is that it is part of the onset of presbyopia. The lens gets harder and less flexible, but also flatter.

For someone with myopia, this means that their refractive error is reduced and thus their distance vision gets better. Unfortunately, it also means that they're going to need longer arms soon.

Appendix

Diopters	Focal Len. (m)	Focal Len. (cm)	Mag. Power
0.25	4	400	1.06
0.50	2	200	1.13
0.75	1.33	133.33	1.19
1.00	1.00	100	1.25
1.25	0.80	80	1.31
1.50	0.67	66.67	1.38
1.75	0.57	57.14	1.44
2.00	0.50	50	1.50
3.00	0.33	33.33	1.75
4.00	0.25	25	2.00
5.00	0.20	20	2.25
6.00	0.17	16.67	2.50
7.00	0.14	14.29	2.75
8.00	0.13	12.5	3.00
9.00	0.11	11.11	3.25
10.00	0.1	10	3.50

Above is a chart that shows the relationship between lens power in diopters to focal length distances. Notice that the difference between say 8.00 and 9.00 diopters is less than 2 centimeters, whereas the difference between 0.75 and 1.00 is more than 33 centimeters.

This is why I call for reductions of whole diopters to start with if you're starting with high-myopia (greater than 6 diopters) and then tapering it off to quarter diopter (0.25) increments.

This is also why I wish I could have had a pair of lenses made with less of a jump when I went from -0.75 to -0.50 because the focal length change was twice that of the one before (first a +33cm jump, then a +66cm jump). A pair of -0.65 lenses would have been perfect.

TREATMENT 3

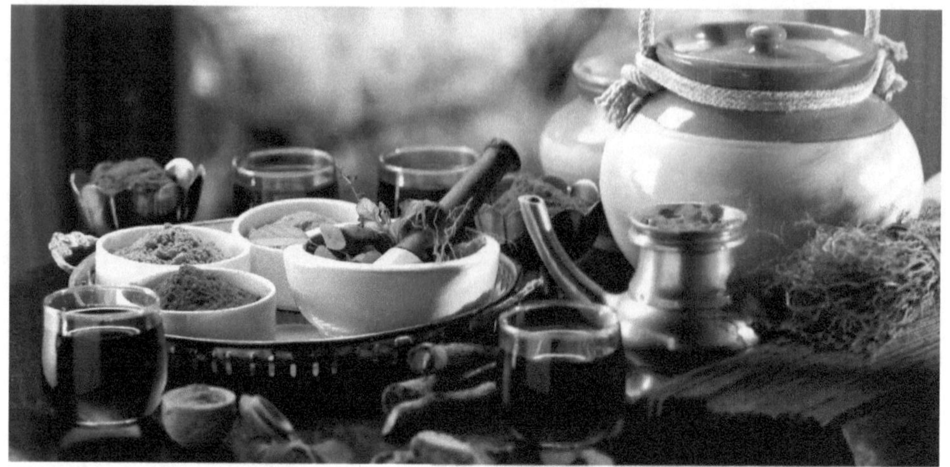

AYURVEDIC

METHOD

Step 1 - Washing Your Eyes

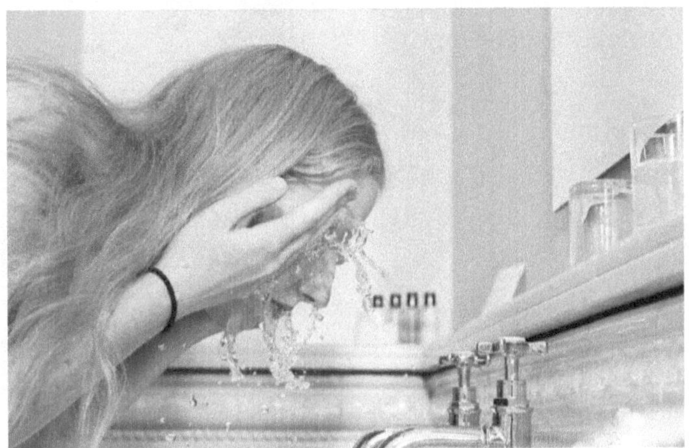

Follow this step early in the morning

Splash Water: Fill mouth with water as it will expand eye muscle properly. Now splash cold water in eyes.

Rose Water: Now use Rosewater to wash your eyes using an eyewash cup.

- Add 10-15 drops of rosewater and rest cold water in an eyewash cup.
- Now place the eyewash cup on one eye and ensure water doesn't spill out from the side.
- Now open your eyes and ensure rose water touch your eye surface, move your pupil in all direction so that water gets circulated properly inside the eye.
- Do this for 1 minute and after that throw away the water and refill the cup in the same way and repeat the same process for the other eye.

These steps will help to calm down inflammation which is the root cause of weak eyesight

Step 2 - Eye Tonic

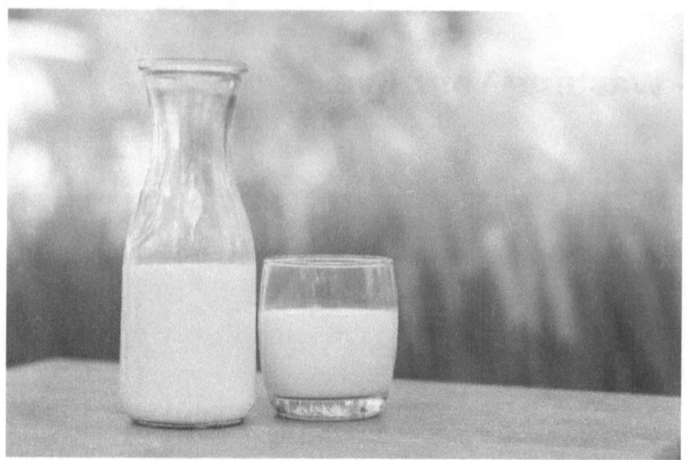

Take this 1 hour before breakfast. This homemade tonic will nourish the nerves of the eyes helping restore lost vision.

- Take 7 soaked and peeled almonds. Don't use California almonds instead use gurbandi almonds (gurbandi almonds are small-sized almonds that are native to the Indian subcontinent and are way more richer in oil, vitamin A, E, and other nutrients that are helpful for the eyes).
- Along with this, you will need 4 whole seeds of black pepper
- Use thread mishri to sweeten it (optional)
- Put all three in the mortar and using the pestle crush them together to form a smooth paste (Mortar and pestle is the traditional way of grinding the medicines. As opposed to a grinder, it does not produce heat and keeps the nutrients intact).
- Now take a pan on low flame and put 1 glass (250ml) of milk (Cow A2 milk) in it, add the paste in it and let the milk boil on low flame for 10 minutes.
- After 10 minutes or so turn off the gas and pour it into a glass. (Do not strain out the mixture).
- Drink this powerful formulation slowly and slowly sip by sip.
- Do not eat anything for the next 1 hour.

Step 3 - Eye Soother

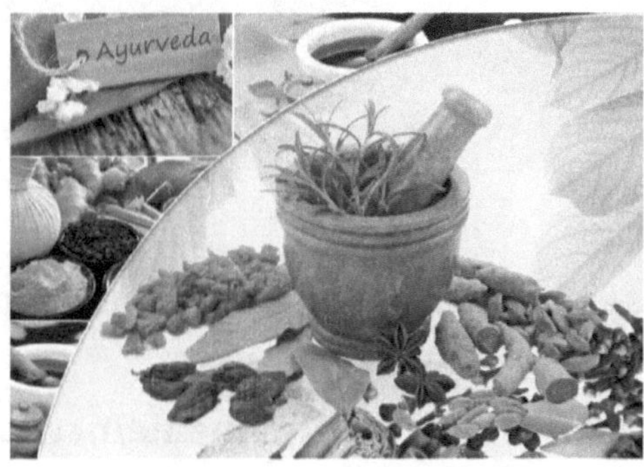

- 30 minutes before going to sleep at night. Take 1 teaspoon mixture of Mahatriphala Ghrit along with 250mg of Abhrak Bhasm, follow this up with one glass of warm milk.

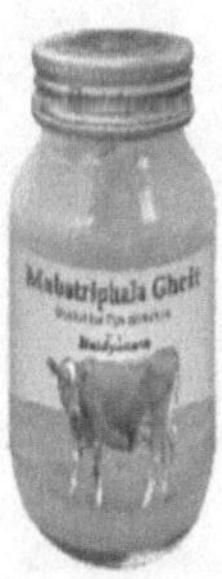

Mahatriphala Ghrit is a combo of ghee along with over a dozen herbs that calm the heat and dryness of eyes)

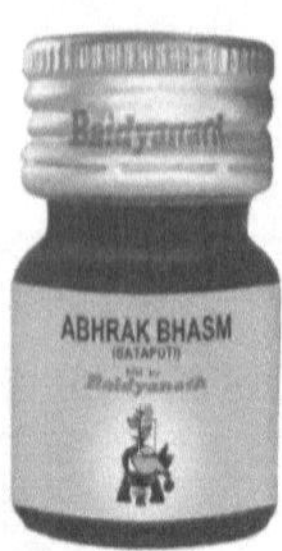

Abhrak Bhasm is a classical Indian medicine prepared from mica and over 60 indigenous herbs)

Both are classical ayurvedic medicines and are highly effective in treating eye disorders.

Step 4 - Optic Massage

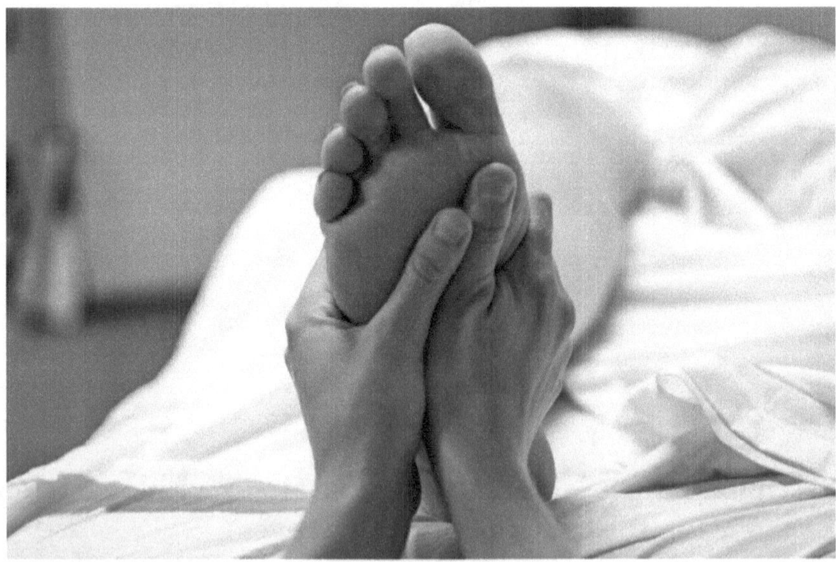

- Just before sleeping, take a few drops of Mahatriphala Ghrit on your hands and massage the soles of your feet. The nerves beneath the soles are directly connected to the optic nerves. This instantly increases blood circulation which helps improve vision.

Step 5 - Mahatriphala Ghrit Eye Drops

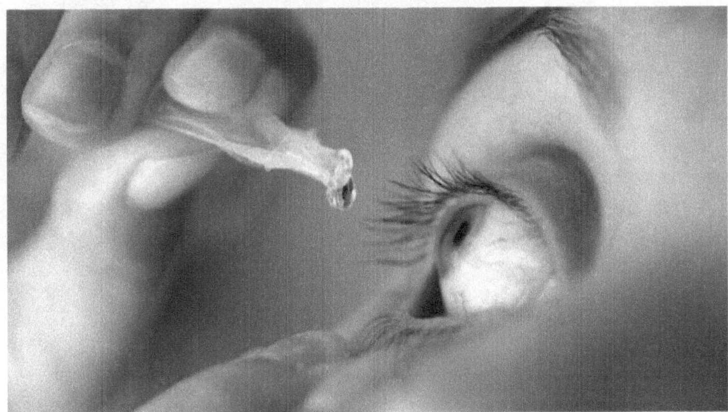

- Finally, the last step is to put a couple of drops of Mahatriphala Ghrit in each of your eyes. Wait about 10 minutes before opening your eye.
- Eyes will go blurry for a while which is normal because that's when you will know that Mahatriphala Ghrit has seeped well into the eyes.

Eye Tonic 2.0 (Can Be Replaced With Step 2)

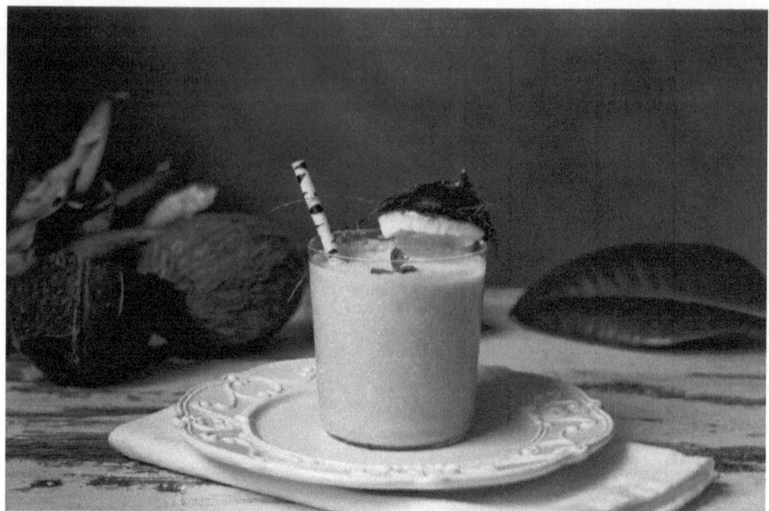

- Take almonds, fennel seeds, and mishri in equal quantity and grind them to make a fine powder.
- Store it in an airtight glass container.
- 30 minutes before going to sleep take 1 tablespoon of this mixture and drink warm milk over it.
- Take this for 3 months.

· **Buying Links**

Rose Water: Link 1 | Link 2

Eye Wash Cup: Link 1 | Link 2

Gurbandi Almonds: Link 1 | Link 2

Black Pepper: Link 1 | Link 2

Thread Mishri: Link 1 | Link 2

Mortar and Pestle: Link 1 | Link 2

Mahatriphala Ghrit: Link 1 | Link 2 | Link 3

Abhrak Bhasm: Link 1 | Link 2

Fennel Seeds: Link 1 | Link 2

If the above links are not working then google the product and you will find them easily.

TREATMENT 4

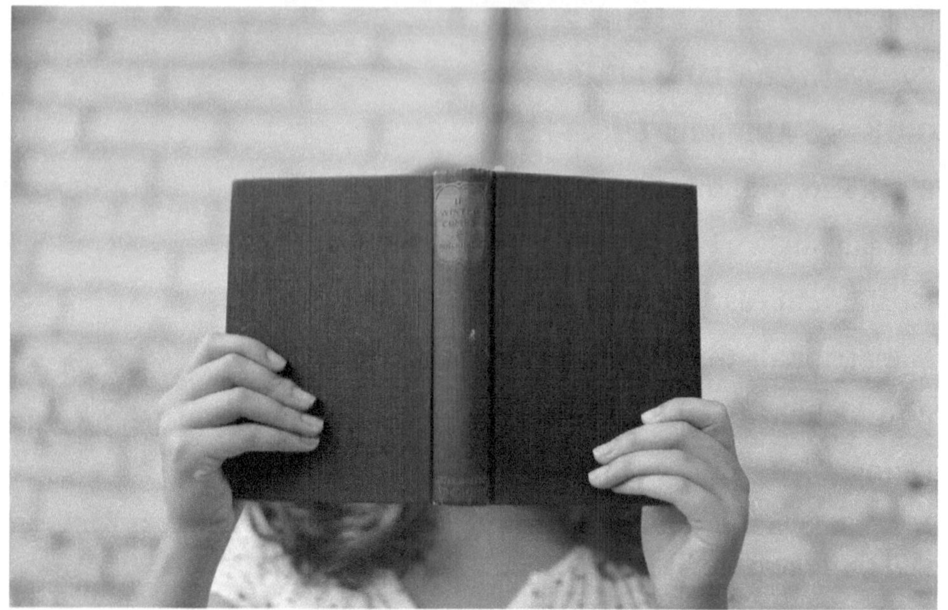

PRINT PUSHING

Print Pushing

Print pushing is the most common name for the practice of placing text at a distance where it just starts to become blurry and then adjusting the distance so that the text goes from blurry to clear.

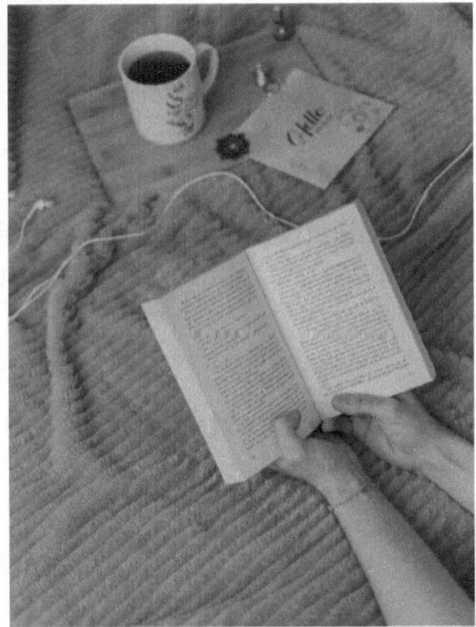

After practicing this, you will notice that the point at which the text becomes blurry is further than it used to be. This is good. Practice print pushing in 15-minute sessions, twice per day but don't try too hard to make the blurry text clearer. This will strain your eyes and make your vision worse.

Step 1: If your myopia is less than -2D, then you will need plus lens and if it more than that you will not need any lens.

Step 2: Get any reading material and keep it at a distance where you can see a little blur.

Step 3: Now try to read it. Blink and you will see that after some time you will be able to read it.

Step 4: Practice this for 15 minutes daily and after some time you will notice that the distance at which you can see clearly increased.

A proper guide to print pushing is given in the below link

https://gettingstronger.org/2016/03/faq-for-vision-improvement-by-hormetism/

How Effective Is Print Pushing?

It is very effective but it will take time to cure Myopia. Don't try too hard otherwise it will strain your eyes. Practice every day for 15-20 minutes 2-3 times. If you want faster results then go for the ancient method.

Video To Learn More About Print Pushing

https://www.youtube.com/watch?v=x5Efg42-Qn0&ab_channel=AncestryFoundation

FAQ

Q: Which treatment is best?

A: Treatment 1 is the best and cheap treatment to cure myopia. It may or may not work for you but if it works then follow it for at least 6 months.

Q: Which treatment to follow first?

A: Why not start all Four. All four treatments are different from one another. Combine all four and follow properly for 3 months and after 3 months get your eyes checked.

Q: Can children below 13 years follow this?

A: Yes, all these methods are very safe. They may or may not work but they will not cause any problem. Actually, vision improvement is very fast in children as compared to adults. You just have to take good care of them. Ensure they don't use mobile phones, make them play outside without glasses so that their eyes can be challenged or if they have high myopia make them use low-powered glasses as discussed in treatment 2.

Q: How long do I have to follow these methods to see visible improvements?

A: Well improvements would be visible in just 1 month. Your eyes will start noticing less strain. Proper reduction in number will be visible in 3 months and major improvements could be visible in 6 months.

Q: My eyes are itching or turning red while following treatment 1.

A: Usually treatment 1 is very safe but if you are experiencing redness or itching then I would request you to stop following the treatment and continue with other treatments.

Q: I can't follow every step mentioned in treatment 3.

A: If you can't follow all steps then you can follow only those with whom you are comfortable. Treatment 3 can be supplemented with other treatments. It will speed the overall healing process. You can implement even one step or all steps from treatment 3 if you are following any other treatment.

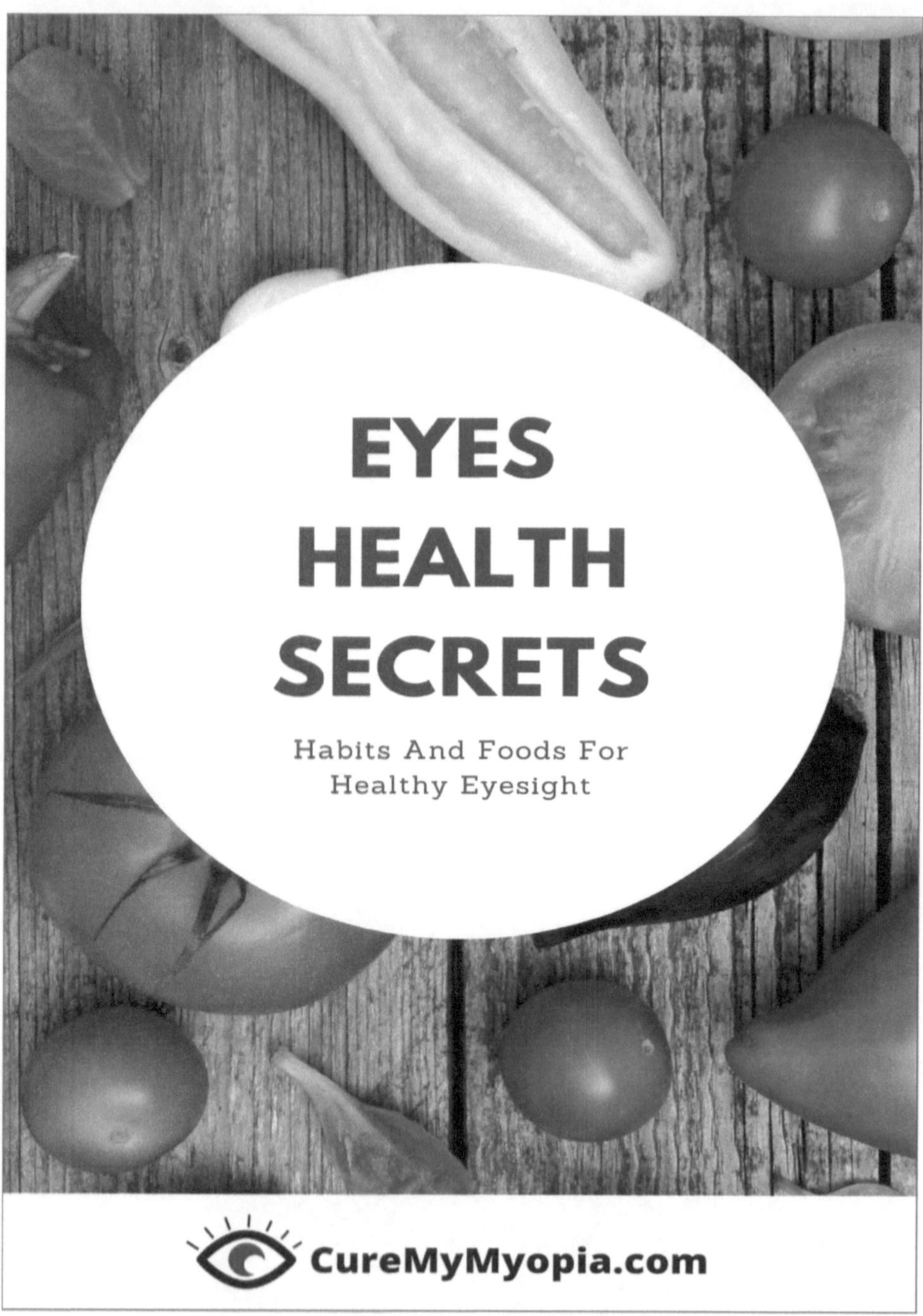
EYES
HEALTH
SECRETS
Habits And Foods For
Healthy Eyesight
CureMyMyopia.com

EYES HEALTH SECRETS

CHAPTER 01

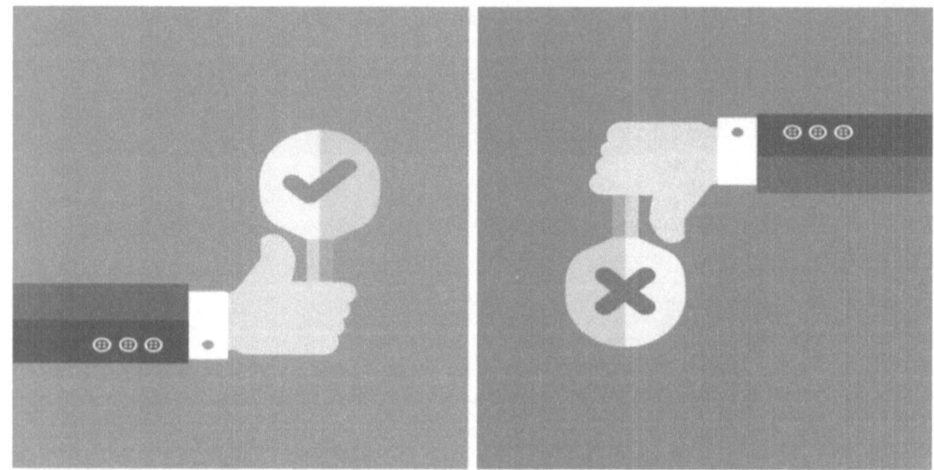

Do's And Don'ts

In the last 10 years, the number of spectacles wearing people increased 4 times. The main reason was watching more computers, mobiles, and T.V screens. When we look at the screen for a long time without blinking, our eyes become dry, and dead skin cells get accumulated at the surface. When more dead cells get accumulated it causes dark circles and eyesight also get weakened.

Do's And Don'ts To Improve Your Eyesight

- Take breaks after every 45 minutes while working and close your eyes for a while and sip some water before getting back to work.
- Rub your palms together and place them over the eyes.
- Press acupressure points whenever you have free time and move your eye around.

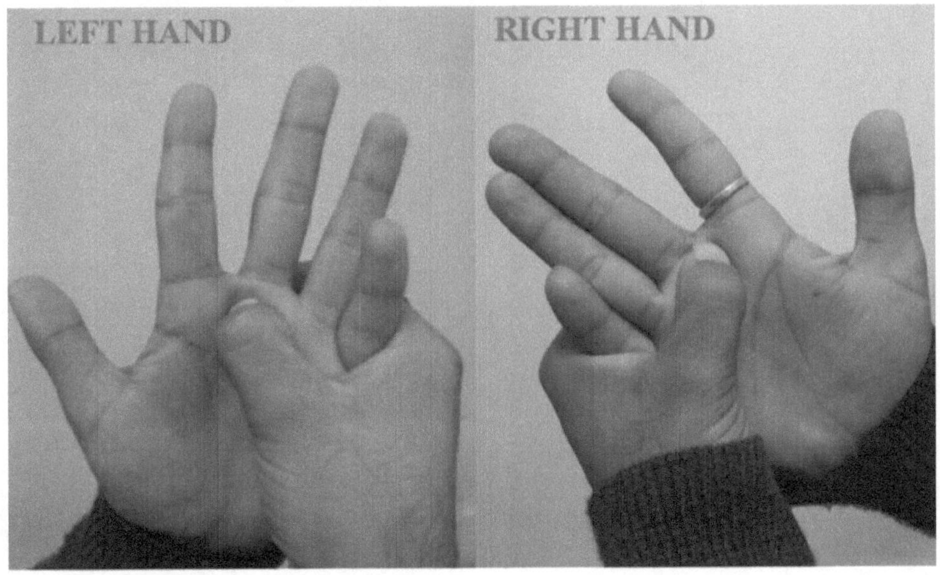

- Every time you go to the washroom. Wash your eyes after filling your mouth with water.
- Avoid walking barefoot as it weakens the eye muscles.
- Blink more often as it prevents drying of eyes.
- Sleep in a dark room and avoid dim lights.
- Protect your eyes from the heat by wearing sunglasses. Sunglasses protect eyes from UV and HEV lights. Prolonged exposure to UV rays can burn cornea which can result in premature aging of eyes and chances of cataract also increases. Wear good quality 100% UV rays-protected sunglasses.
- Use a screen guard on screens to protect your eyes.
- Practice Sarvangasana as it increases blood circulation to your eyes.

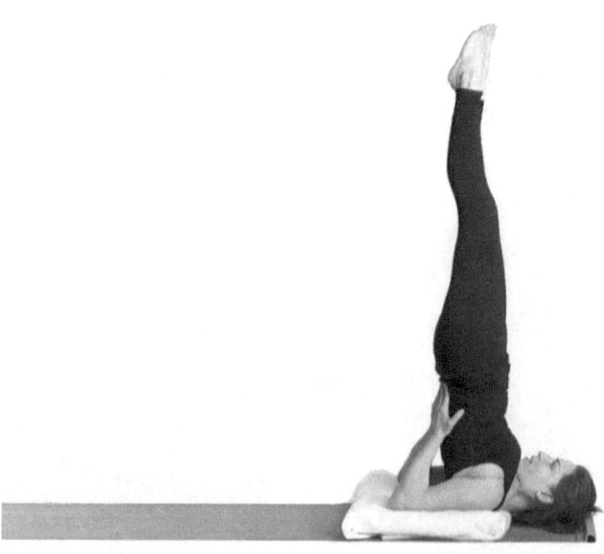

- Don't rub your eyes as eyes are very delicate and rubbing them will seriously damage the eye blood vessels.
- If there is an itch, then gently use your fingers to calm it down.

- Don't read while traveling as the text is not stable which causes constant strain on the eyes and the eyes find it hard to focus on the text.
- Tiny letters on the phone also cause strain on the eye.
- Don't use dim light to study. Avoid studying in low light.
- Reading or writing in low light causes strain on the eyes muscles which weaken eyes muscles.
- Never use mobile with room lights off as eyes will get weak very rapidly. Use proper lighting.
- Practice eye exercises for 3-5 minutes daily like moving your eyeballs in a circular motion.
- Tightly close your eyes, hold for 3 seconds and open.
- Rub your palms together place them on your eyes (the warmth will relax the eye muscles).
- Walking barefoot on grass early in the morning and looking at natural greenery soothes the eye.

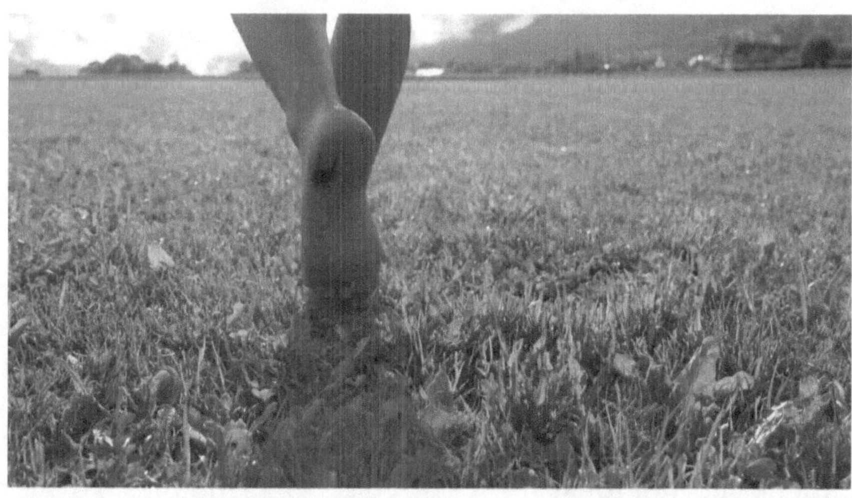

Habits That Destroys Your Eyesight

NOT USING SUNGLASSES

The UV rays from the sun can damage the eyes. You should always wear UV-protective sunglasses or glasses when outside even on a cloudy day.

DRINKING ALCOHOL

Too much alcohol can cause problems for your eyes. Alcohol can cause eye conditions to develop sooner, like macular degeneration. Try to limit your alcohol intake.

TOO MUCH SCREEN TIME

Nowadays people spend a huge amount of their time using smartphones, computers, TVs, and other screen devices. The devices can cause eyes to dry and can even cause eye strain which can lead to a decrease in vision and ultimately result in Myopia.

OVERUSING EYE DROPS

Eye drops that promise to remove redness from the eyes are not good for your eyesight. These types of eye drops can restrict blood flow in the eyes and can cause damages to your eyes.

EYEGLASSES

Having myopia in which a person can't see the distant object clearly and using the eyeglasses even for close distant can worsen your eyesight. If your distant vision is poor then why use glasses for closer distance. Myopia glasses are meant to be used for seeing distant objects not for seeing close objects like mobiles. This is the main reason why your glasses number increases year by year.

CONTACT LENSES

The same concept applies to contact lenses also. They are meant to be used for seeing at distance, not for close work. Contact lenses also dry your eyes and there is a risk of some type of eye infection.

SMOKING

Smoking generally has a wide range of health issues. The smoke can burn your eyes and the chemicals that are used in tobacco products have serious side effects on eyesight which can even cause a cataract at a younger age.

RUBBING YOUR EYES

Itchy eyes are very annoying but rubbing your eyes can make the problem worse. Rubbing can put unnecessary pressure on your eyes.

NOT EATING PROPER DIET

Eating a balanced diet is very important for your eyes. Our eyes need vitamins and nutrients to stay healthy. Include foods that are rich in vitamin C, Zinc, Vitamin E, and Omega-3 fatty acids. A complete list of food items that help with vision is given in Chapter 2.

NOT SLEEPING PROPERLY

Sleeping less can cause vision problems. It can cause red, puffy, or itchy eyes. Try to get at least 7 hours of sleep. Take a break from the screen at least 1 hour before sleeping otherwise it will interfere with your sleep cycle.

USING SCREEN IN DARK

Using mobiles, TV, or other screen devices in dark is not recommended. It can put a lot of strain on your eyes and eventually can result in vision loss in the long run. So, avoid using phones or other devices in dark.

CONSTIPATION

Have you ever noticed that your vision is a lot poor when you are constipated? Having constipation can seriously impact your eyesight. So, try to sleep on time and eat a healthy fibrous diet.

STRESS

Stress has a lot of health issues. Be it mental or physical. Too much stress can weaken eyesight. Try to avoid stress as much as possible. Do some meditation or Yoga. One of the methods that I find very helpful for overcoming stress is Wim Hoff Method. Search for it on YouTube.

Habits That Improves Eyesight

ACTIVE FOCUS

It is single handily one of the best practices, methods, or exercises to cure vision problems. What you have to do is challenge your vision. You have to voluntarily control your vision. It is not hard to do and you can do it any time of the day.

You have to introduce some blur and voluntarily try to get things in focus. Suppose you are watching TV. Remove your glasses or if you have high Myopia use glasses that are not that much powerful (Refer to vision improvement secrets). Now look at the TV and try to make what is on the TV. Blink and you will notice that after some time you can see clearly what is on the TV.

This is called Active Focus.

Refer to https://endmyopia.org/active-focus-links to get full knowledge about active focus. It is a great website with a lot of scientific proof.

SEEING GREENERY

Seeing greenery soothes the eyes. Take out some time from your busy schedule and go for a walk where you can look at greenery. It will be very refreshing for your eyes. Try to avoid your glasses and practice Active Focus.

WALKING BAREFOOTED ON GRASS

Walking barefoot on grasses early in the morning helps with vision. Walking also improves overall health. Remember to only walk barefoot on grass otherwise, your eyesight will decrease.

WATCHING TV WITHOUT GLASSES

As absurd as it sounds but TV can help with your vision. Watch TV without wearing your glasses and practice Active Focus. Initially, you will have some problems. Try to get used to the blur vision. By doing Active Focus you can easily watch TV. It will be also a good exercise.

MEDITATION

Meditation helps to reduce stress and also relaxes the body. It will be of great help to your eyes. Practice meditation for at least 15 minutes daily.

EATING HEALTHY FRUITS AND VEGETABLES

Eating fruits and vegetables is very good for your eyes. Eat green vegetables and drink some juice. Never depends on multivitamins tablets as they are not easily absorbed by the body. There are scientific studies that proofs that multivitamins tablets are not effective. There is no substitute for fruits and vegetables. Eat only natural and avoid processed foods as they lack nutrients.

CHAPTER 02

DIET

C arrots may be the food best known for helping your eyes. But other foods and their nutrients may be more important for keeping your eyesight keen as you age.

Vitamin C and E, zinc, lutein, zeaxanthin, and omega -3 fatty acids all play a role in eye health. They can help prevent the clouding of your eye lens. They also fight the most likely cause of vision loss when you're older. "It's always best to get the nutrients we know help vision from foods".

Some Powerhouse Foods For Healthy Eyes To Try.

Spinach and Kale: Antioxidants protect against eye damage from things like sunlight, cigarette smoke, and air pollution. These leafy greens are loaded with two of the best for eyes, lutein, and zeaxanthin.

"They get into the lens and retina of your eye, and they are believed to absorb damaging visible light,"

Most people are short on these two nutrients.

Oranges, Carrots, Strawberries, etc: Vitamin C is a top antioxidant. These foods are among the top sources of vitamin C. Eat strawberries (one-half cup) a day and you're good to go. Papaya, oranges, and green peppers are other good sources.

Seeds and Nuts: Vitamin C and E work together to keep healthy tissue strong. But most of us don't get as much Vitamin E as we should be getting from food. Have a small handful of sunflower seeds. Almonds, pecans, and vegetable oils are also good sources. Omega 3 rich foods like soaked walnuts, flaxseeds, salmon are essential for the eyes.

Amla (Indian Gooseberry): Consume one amla a day as it is excellent for the eyes. They are very rich in Vitamin C which is very essential for the eyes.

Eye strengthening Foods: Consume eye strengthening foods like ghee (Clarified Butter), Moong Dal 2-3 times a week.

Green Leafy Vegetables: All green leafy vegetables are rich in zeaxanthin and lutein which are the two most important nutrients for the eyes.

Salt: Cut down salt intake as it dehydrates the eyes.

FOODS FOR BETTER EYESIGHT

NUTS AND LEGUMES

They are rich in omega-3 fatty acids and are also high in vitamin E which protects the eye from age-related damage.

- Walnuts
- Brazil Nuts
- Cashews
- Peanuts
- Lentils

SEEDS

Seeds are also high in omega 3 and vitamin E

- Chia seeds
- Flax seeds
- Hemp seeds

CITRUS FRUITS

They are rich in Vitamin C which is an antioxidant

- Lemons

- Oranges
- Grapefruits

GREEN LEAFY VEGETABLES

Rich in lutein and zeaxanthin

- Spinach
- Kale
- Collards

CARROTS

Rich in vitamin A and Beta Carotene. Vitamin A plays an essential role in vision. It is a component of a protein called rhodopsin, which helps to absorb light.

SWEET POTATOES

They are also rich in beta carotene. They are also rich in Vitamin E.

TRIPHALA

Triphala is a herbal formula that is made up of three fruits – Amla, Bibhitaki, and Haritaki. It has strong medicinal properties and is widely used in Ayurvedic Medicines to lower toxicity levels in the body. It is also very good for eyesight.

CREDITS

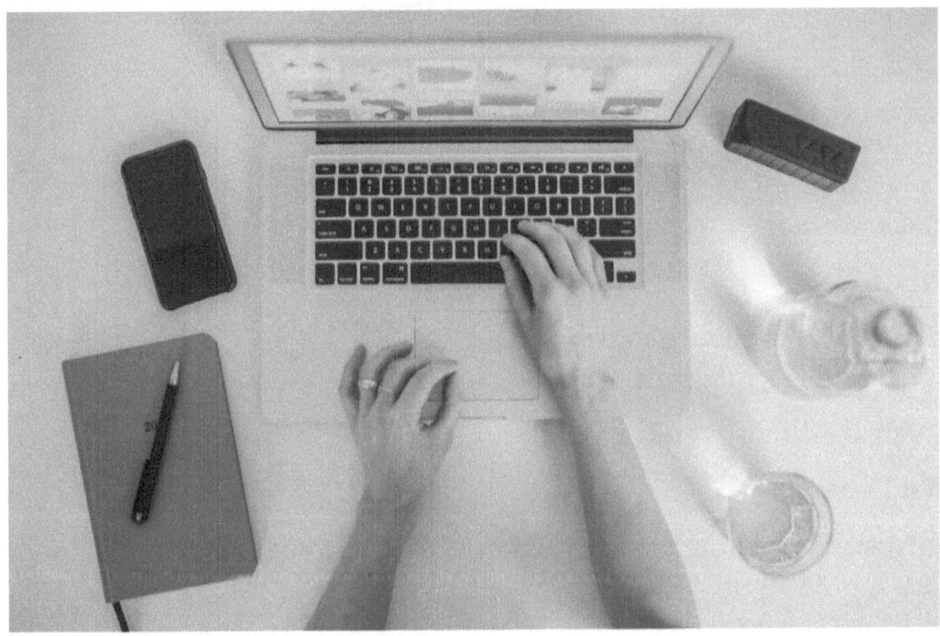

Introduction And Treatment 02

The No Bulls#*t Guide to Vision Improvement By C.G. Hayes

https://www.youtube.com/user/cliffgnu

Special Thanks

Jake Steiner

Youtube :

https://www.youtube.com/channel/
UCEhYxefHylpSgoiXDWcBrlA

Website: https://endmyopia.org/

FitTuber

https://www.youtube.com/channel/UCYC6Vcczj8v-
Y5OgpEJTFBw

FEEDBACK

We would love to hear your experience and feedback after using our guide. If you have seen any visible improvement or have any other method that could benefit others then kindly share it with us.

Website: https://www.curemymyopia.com

Email: info@beinghealthysutra.com

9 798491 660032